CELIAC DISEASE COOKBOOK FOR KIDS

Nutritious and Easy-to-Make Gluten-Free Meal Plans for Happy and Healthier Kids

Sonia Emmason

Copyright © 2023 by Sonia Emmason

CHAPTER 1

Celiac disease is a genetic autoimmune disorder that affects millions of people worldwide, including children. This condition is caused by the body's inability to tolerate gluten, a protein found in wheat, barley, and rye. When people with celiac disease consume gluten, their immune system responds by attacking the small intestine, which can lead to a range of symptoms such as abdominal pain, bloating, diarrhea, fatigue, and nutrient deficiencies.

The best treatment for celiac disease is a strict gluten-free diet, which involves avoiding all foods and beverages that contain gluten. This can be a challenging task, especially for children who often have limited food choices and may not fully understand the impact of their diet on their health. However, with the right guidance and support, it is possible for children with celiac disease to enjoy a healthy and delicious gluten-free diet.

The purpose of this cookbook is to provide parents, caregivers, and children with practical tips and tasty recipes to help them navigate the challenges of a celiac disease diet. This cookbook is designed to be kid-friendly and easy to use, with step-by-step instructions and that will appeal to young readers.

The recipes in this cookbook have been carefully selected to provide a balanced and nutritious diet that meets the unique needs of children with celiac disease. All of the recipes are gluten-free and have been taste-tested by kids to ensure they are delicious and appealing. The cookbook includes a variety of recipes for breakfast, lunch, dinner, and snacks.

One of the most challenging aspects of a celiac disease diet is the need to avoid gluten while still ensuring that children receive all the essential nutrients they need for healthy growth and development. Gluten-free foods are often lower in fiber, vitamins, and minerals than their gluten-containing counterparts, which can put children at risk for nutrient deficiencies.

However, by choosing nutrient-dense gluten-free foods such as fruits, vegetables, lean proteins, and whole grains such as quinoa, buckwheat, and amaranth, parents can help their children maintain a healthy and balanced diet.

A celiac disease diet can be challenging, but with the right guidance and support, children with celiac disease can thrive and enjoy a healthy and delicious gluten-free diet.

CHAPTER 2

Celiac disease is a chronic autoimmune disorder that affects the small intestine of children and adults. It is caused by an immune response to gluten, a protein found in wheat, barley, and rye. When gluten is consumed, it triggers an abnormal immune response in people with celiac disease, leading to inflammation and damage to the lining of the small intestine.

Celiac disease can manifest in a variety of ways, and symptoms can vary widely from person to person. In children, symptoms may include abdominal pain, bloating, diarrhea, constipation, vomiting, and weight loss. However, some children with celiac disease may have no symptoms at all, making it difficult to diagnose.

If left untreated, celiac disease can lead to serious health consequences, including malnutrition, anemia, osteoporosis, and an increased risk of other autoimmune disorders, such as type 1 diabetes and thyroid disease.

For this reason, it is important for children who are suspected of having celiac disease to receive an accurate diagnosis and timely treatment.

The diagnosis of celiac disease in children typically involves a combination of blood tests and a biopsy of the small intestine. Blood tests can detect the presence of antibodies that are produced when the body reacts to gluten. If these tests are positive, a biopsy is usually performed to confirm the diagnosis and assess the extent of damage to the small intestine.

The best treatment for celiac disease is a strict gluten-free diet, which involves avoiding all foods and beverages that contain gluten. This can be challenging for children, who may feel left out or different from their peers. It is important for parents and caregivers to provide emotional support and practical guidance to help children adjust to the gluten-free diet.

A gluten-free diet can also pose nutritional challenges, as gluten-free foods are often lower in fiber, vitamins, and minerals than their gluten-containing counterparts.

In addition to following a gluten-free diet, children with celiac disease may need to be monitored regularly by a healthcare provider to assess their growth and nutritional status. They may also need to undergo periodic blood tests to check for nutrient deficiencies and to ensure that the gluten-free diet is being followed effectively.

Celiac disease is a chronic autoimmune disorder that can have serious health consequences if left untreated. It is important for parents and caregivers to be aware of the symptoms of celiac disease in children and to seek medical attention if there are concerns. With proper diagnosis, treatment, and nutritional support, children with celiac disease can lead healthy and active lives.

CHAPTER 3

STOCKING A GLUTEN-FREE KITCHEN

Stocking a gluten-free kitchen can be a challenge, but with a little bit of planning and organization, it is possible to create a safe and delicious environment for people with celiac disease or gluten intolerance. Here are some tips for stocking a gluten-free kitchen:

1. **Start with a thorough cleaning:** Before stocking your kitchen with gluten-free items, it is important to clean all surfaces, utensils, and appliances to remove any traces of gluten. This includes wiping down countertops, washing dishes and cookware, and cleaning out your pantry and refrigerator.

2. **Separate gluten-free items from gluten-containing items:** Once your kitchen is clean, it is important to keep gluten-free items separate from gluten-containing items. This can be done by designating specific shelves or cabinets for gluten-free foods, using different colored labels

for gluten-free items, and using separate utensils for cooking and preparing gluten-free meals.

3. **Stock up on gluten-free staples:** Some gluten-free staples to have on hand include gluten-free flours (such as rice, potato, and corn flour), gluten-free pasta, gluten-free bread, and gluten-free snacks (such as crackers and chips). These items can be found at most grocery stores, health food stores, or online.

4. **Use fresh ingredients:** Fresh fruits, vegetables, and meats are naturally gluten-free and are a great way to add flavor and nutrition to your gluten-free meals. By using fresh ingredients, you can avoid the need for gluten-containing seasonings or sauces.

5. **Read labels carefully:** When shopping for packaged foods, it is important to read labels carefully to ensure that they are gluten-free. Look for products that are labeled "gluten-free" or "certified gluten-free", and avoid foods that contain wheat, barley, rye, or malt.

6. **Consider cross-contamination:** Even small amounts of gluten can be harmful to people with celiac disease or gluten intolerance. To avoid cross-contamination, use separate cutting boards, utensils, and cookware for gluten-free meals, and avoid using shared appliances such as toasters or fryers.

By following these tips, you can create a safe and delicious gluten-free kitchen for people with celiac disease or gluten intolerance. With a little bit of planning and organization, you can enjoy gluten-free meals that are healthy and delicious.

CHAPTER 3

Cooking and baking can be a fun and rewarding experience, especially when preparing gluten-free meals and desserts for those with celiac disease or gluten intolerance. Here are some cooking and baking basics to keep in mind when preparing gluten-free foods:

1. **Use gluten-free ingredients:** When cooking or baking gluten-free, it is important to use ingredients that are naturally gluten-free or labeled as gluten-free. This includes flours, grains, and starches such as rice flour, almond flour, quinoa, and cornstarch. Be sure to check labels to ensure that ingredients are gluten-free.

2. **Adjust recipes:** Many traditional recipes can be adapted to be gluten-free by substituting gluten-free flours and ingredients. Keep in mind that gluten-free flours may require different amounts of liquid or different cooking times, so be prepared to experiment with recipe adjustments.

3. **Use gluten-free seasonings and sauces:** Many seasonings and sauces may contain gluten, so it is important to read labels and look for products that are labeled as gluten-free. Alternatively, consider making your own gluten-free seasonings and sauces using fresh herbs, spices, and gluten-free ingredients.

4. **Be mindful of cross-contamination:** Even small amounts of gluten can cause a reaction in people with celiac disease or gluten intolerance. To avoid cross-contamination, use separate utensils, cutting boards, and cookware for gluten-free meals, and thoroughly clean all surfaces and appliances before preparing gluten-free foods.

5. **Experiment with new recipes:** There are many delicious gluten-free recipes available online or in cookbooks. Experiment with new recipes to find ones that you enjoy, and adapt your favorite recipes to be gluten-free.

6. **Consider texture and consistency:** Gluten-free flours and ingredients may have different textures and consistencies than their gluten-

containing counterparts. Consider the texture and consistency of the ingredients when adapting recipes, and be prepared to experiment with recipe adjustments to achieve the desired texture and consistency.

7. **Practice food safety:** As with any type of cooking or baking, it is important to practice food safety when preparing gluten-free foods. This includes washing hands and utensils thoroughly, cooking foods to the appropriate temperature, and refrigerating foods promptly.

By keeping these cooking and baking basics in mind, you can prepare delicious gluten-free meals and desserts that are safe and enjoyable for people with celiac disease or gluten intolerance. With a little bit of experimentation and creativity, you can create meals and treats that are both healthy and delicious.

CHAPTER 4

4.0 Healthy Celiac Disease Recipes for kids

4.1 DELICIOUS BREAKFASTS

1. Gluten-Free Banana Pancakes (15 minutes)

Ingredients:

- ½ cup gluten-free flour

- 1 teaspoon baking powder

- ½ teaspoon ground cinnamon

- ¼ teaspoon salt

- 1 egg

- ¾ cup almond milk

- 1 tablespoon melted butter

- 1 mashed banana

Instructions:

1. In a medium bowl, whisk together the flour, baking powder, cinnamon, and salt.

2. In a separate bowl, whisk together the egg, almond milk, and melted butter.

3. Add the wet ingredients to the dry ingredients and mix until combined.

4. Heat a griddle or pan over medium heat and spray with non-stick cooking spray.

5. Pour ¼ cup of batter onto the hot griddle and cook until bubbles form and the edges are golden brown.

6. Flip the pancake and cook until the other side is golden brown.

7. Repeat with the remaining batter.

8. Serve with desired toppings.

Ingredients:

- 4 eggs

- 4 slices of gluten-free bread

- 4 slices of cooked bacon

- 4 tablespoons of shredded cheese

- Salt and pepper to taste

Instructions:

1. Preheat oven to 350°F.

2. Grease a muffin tin with non-stick cooking spray.

3. Place a slice of bread in each muffin cup and press down to fit.

4. Place a slice of bacon in each muffin cup.

5. Crack an egg into each muffin cup and season with salt and pepper.

6. Sprinkle with shredded cheese.

7. Bake for 15 minutes or until eggs are set.

8. Serve warm.

Ingredients:

- 4 slices of gluten-free bread

- 2 eggs

- ¼ cup almond milk

- 1 teaspoon ground cinnamon

- 2 tablespoons melted butter

Instructions:

1. Preheat oven to 350°F.

2. Cut the bread into strips.

3. In a shallow bowl, whisk together the eggs, almond milk, and cinnamon.

4. Dip the bread strips in the egg mixture, coating both sides.

5. Place the bread strips on a baking sheet lined with parchment paper.

6. Drizzle the melted butter over the bread strips.

7. Bake for 15 minutes or until golden brown.

8. Serve warm with maple syrup.

Ingredients:

- ½ cup rolled oats

- ½ cup almond milk

- 2 tablespoons chia seeds

- 1 teaspoon honey

- ½ teaspoon ground cinnamon

- ¼ teaspoon vanilla extract

Instructions:

1. In a bowl, combine the oats, almond milk, chia seeds, honey, cinnamon, and vanilla extract.

2. Mix until combined.

3. Cover the bowl and place in the fridge overnight.

4. Serve cold or warm in the morning.

Ingredients:

- 2 cups gluten-free rolled oats

- 1 teaspoon baking powder

- ½ teaspoon ground cinnamon

- ½ teaspoon salt

- 2 eggs

- 1 cup almond milk

- ¼ cup maple syrup

- 2 tablespoons melted butter

- 1 teaspoon vanilla extract

Instructions:

1. Preheat oven to 350°F.

2. Grease an 8"x8" baking pan with non-stick cooking spray.

3. In a medium bowl, whisk together the oats, baking powder, cinnamon, and salt.

4. In a separate bowl, whisk together the eggs, almond milk, maple syrup, melted butter, and vanilla extract.

5. Add the wet ingredients to the dry ingredients and mix until combined.

6. Pour the oatmeal mixture into the greased baking pan.

7. Bake for 40-45 minutes or until golden brown.

8. Serve with desired toppings.

Ingredients:

- 1 cup gluten-free flour

- 1 teaspoon baking powder

- ½ teaspoon ground cinnamon

- ¼ teaspoon salt

- 2 eggs

- 1 cup almond milk

- 2 tablespoons melted butter

- 1 teaspoon vanilla extract

Instructions:

1. Preheat waffle iron.

2. In a medium bowl, whisk together the flour, baking powder, cinnamon, and salt.

3. In a separate bowl, whisk together the eggs, almond milk, melted butter, and vanilla extract.

4. Add the wet ingredients to the dry ingredients and mix until combined.

5. Pour the batter into the preheated waffle iron and cook until golden brown.

6. Serve with desired toppings.

Ingredients:

- 1 cup frozen berries

- ½ banana

- 1 cup almond milk

- 2 tablespoons gluten-free protein powder

- 1 tablespoon honey

- Toppings of your choice

Instructions:

1. Place all ingredients in a blender and blend until smooth.

2. Pour into a bowl and top with desired toppings.

3. Serve immediately.

Ingredients:

- 1 cup gluten-free flour

- 1 teaspoon baking powder

- ½ teaspoon ground cinnamon

- ¼ teaspoon salt

- 2 eggs

- ½ cup almond milk

- ¼ cup melted butter

- 1 teaspoon vanilla extract

- ½ cup chopped nuts

Instructions:

1. Preheat oven to 350°F.

2. Grease a 12-cup muffin tin with non-stick cooking spray.

3. In a medium bowl, whisk together the flour, baking powder, cinnamon, and salt.

4. In a separate bowl, whisk together the eggs, almond milk, melted butter, and vanilla extract.

5. Add the wet ingredients to the dry ingredients and mix until combined.

6. Fold in the chopped nuts.

7. Divide the batter evenly among the muffin cups.

8. Bake for 15 minutes or until golden brown.

9. Serve warm.

9. Egg and Cheese Wrap (10 minutes)

Ingredients:

- 1 gluten-free tortilla

- 2 eggs

- 2 tablespoons shredded cheese

- Salt and pepper to taste

Instructions:

1. Heat a skillet over medium heat.

2. Spray the skillet with non-stick cooking spray.

3. Crack the eggs into the skillet and season with salt and pepper.

4. Cook until the eggs are set.

5. Place the eggs on the tortilla and top with shredded cheese.

6. Roll the tortilla up and serve warm.

Ingredients:

- 1 gluten-free bagel

- 2 tablespoons cream cheese

- Toppings of your choice

Instructions:

1. Toast the gluten-free bagel.

2. Spread the cream cheese on the bagel.

3. Top with desired toppings.

4. Serve warm.

1. Gluten-Free Cheese Crackers (10 minutes)

Ingredients:

- 1/2 cup of gluten-free flour

- 1/2 cup of grated cheddar cheese

Instructions:

1. Preheat the oven to 350°F.

2. In a bowl, mix together the gluten-free flour and grated cheddar cheese.

3. On a lightly floured surface, roll out the dough until it is 1/4-inch thick.

4. Cut out small crackers with a cookie cutter, or use a knife to cut them into desired shapes.

5. Place the crackers on a lightly greased baking sheet.

6. Bake for 10 minutes, or until the crackers are golden brown.

7. Allow to cool before serving.

Ingredients:

- Your favorite fruits, cut into bite-sized pieces

- 1/4 cup of unsweetened applesauce

Instructions:

1. Thread the fruit pieces onto skewers.

2. Place the kabobs onto a plate or cutting board.

3. Drizzle the applesauce over the kabobs and serve.

Ingredients:

- 2 medium sweet potatoes, cut into wedges

- 1 tablespoon of olive oil

- 1 teaspoon of garlic powder

- 1 teaspoon of paprika

- Salt and pepper to taste

Instructions:

1. Preheat the oven to 425°F.

2. Place the sweet potato wedges on a baking sheet.

3. Drizzle with olive oil and sprinkle with garlic powder, paprika, salt and pepper.

4. Bake for 15-20 minutes, or until the sweet potatoes are golden brown and cooked through.

5. Serve with your favorite dipping sauce.

Ingredients:

- 1 cup of cooked quinoa

- 1/2 cup of shredded carrots

- 1/2 cup of corn

- 1/2 cup of peas

- 1/2 cup of grated cheese

- 2 eggs

- 1/4 cup of gluten-free breadcrumbs

- Salt and pepper to taste

Instructions:

1. Preheat the oven to 375°F.

2. In a large bowl, combine the quinoa, carrots, corn, peas, cheese, eggs, breadcrumbs and salt and pepper.

3. Mix until everything is combined.

4. Form the mixture into small balls and place them on a greased baking sheet.

5. Bake for 20-25 minutes, or until the bites are golden brown.

6. Serve warm with your favorite dipping sauce.

Ingredients:

- 2 cups of grated zucchini

- 1/2 cup of gluten-free flour

- 2 eggs

- 2 tablespoons of grated Parmesan cheese

- 1 teaspoon of garlic powder

- Salt and pepper to taste

Instructions:

1. In a bowl, combine the zucchini, gluten-free flour, eggs, Parmesan cheese, garlic powder, salt and pepper.

2. Mix until everything is well combined.

3. Heat a large skillet over medium heat.

4. Drop spoonful of the zucchini mixture into the skillet and cook for 3-4 minutes per side, or until the fritters are golden brown.

5. Serve warm with your favorite dipping sauce.

Ingredients:

- 3 large carrots, cut into matchsticks

- 1 tablespoon of olive oil

- 1 teaspoon of garlic powder

- 1 teaspoon of paprika

- Salt and pepper to taste

Instructions:

1. Preheat the oven to 400°F.

2. Place the carrot matchsticks on a baking sheet.

3. Drizzle with olive oil and sprinkle with garlic powder, paprika, salt and pepper.

4. Bake for 25-30 minutes, or until the carrots are golden brown and cooked through.

5. Serve warm with your favorite dipping sauce.

Ingredients:

- 2 slices of gluten-free bread

- 1 ripe avocado, pitted and mashed

- 1 teaspoon of lime juice

- Salt and pepper to taste

Instructions:

1. Toast the gluten-free bread in a toaster or under the broiler.

2. In a bowl, mash the avocado with the lime juice, salt and pepper.

3. Spread the mashed avocado onto the toast.

4. Serve immediately.

Ingredients:

- 1 package of gluten-free pizza dough

- 1/2 cup of shredded mozzarella cheese

- 1/4 cup of pizza sauce

Instructions:

1. Preheat the oven to 375°F.

2. On a lightly floured surface, roll out the pizza dough into a 9x13-inch rectangle.

3. Spread the pizza sauce over the dough and sprinkle with the cheese.

4. Roll the dough up into a log and cut into 1-inch slices.

5. Place the slices on a lightly greased baking sheet.

6. Bake for 20-25 minutes, or until the rolls are golden brown.

7. Serve warm with additional pizza sauce for dipping.

Ingredients:

- 1 apple, cored and thinly sliced

- 2 tablespoons of peanut butter

- 2 tablespoons of gluten-free granola

- 2 tablespoons of chocolate chips

Instructions:

1. Place the apple slices on a plate.

2. Spread the peanut butter over the apple slices.

3. Sprinkle the granola and chocolate chips over the apple slices.

4. Serve immediately.

Ingredients:

- 1 cup of plain yogurt

- 1/4 cup of gluten-free granola

- 1/4 cup of fresh berries

Instructions:

1. In a bowl or parfait glass, layer the yogurt, granola and berries.

2. Serve immediately.

4.3 SOUPS AND SALADS

1. Creamy Potato Soup (40 minutes)

Ingredients:

- 2 tablespoons of butter

- 1 medium onion, diced

- 2 cloves of garlic, minced

- 5 cups of gluten-free chicken or vegetable stock

- 4 large potatoes, peeled and diced

- 1 cup of cream

- Salt and freshly ground black pepper, to taste

Instructions:

1. Melt butter in a large pot over medium heat.

2. Add the onion and garlic and cook until softened, about 5 minutes.

3. Add the stock, potatoes, and season with salt and pepper.

4. Bring to a boil, then reduce heat and simmer until potatoes are tender, about 25 minutes.

5. Puree the soup with an immersion blender until smooth.

6. Stir in cream, and season with salt and pepper, to taste.

7. Serve hot.

Ingredients:

- 2 tablespoons of olive oil

- 1 medium onion, diced

- 2 cloves of garlic, minced

- 2 red bell peppers, seeded and diced

- 4 cups of gluten-free chicken or vegetable stock

- 1 teaspoon of smoked paprika

- 1 teaspoon of cumin

- Salt and freshly ground black pepper, to taste

- 1/2 cup of cream

Instructions:

1. Preheat oven to 400F.

2. Place the bell peppers on a baking sheet, and roast for 25 minutes, until softened and charred.

3. Heat the oil in a large pot over medium heat.

4. Add the onion and garlic, and cook until softened, about 5 minutes.

5. Add the roasted bell peppers, stock, paprika, and cumin.

6. Bring to a boil, then reduce heat and simmer for 20 minutes.

7. Puree the soup with an immersion blender until smooth.

8. Stir in cream, and season with salt and pepper, to taste.

9. Serve hot.

Ingredients:

- 1 cup of quinoa

- 2 tablespoons of olive oil

- 2 cloves of garlic, minced

- 2 cups of water

- 1/2 cup of fresh parsley, chopped

- 1/2 cup of fresh mint, chopped

- 1/2 cup of fresh tomatoes, diced

- 1/4 cup of fresh lemon juice

- Salt and freshly ground black pepper, to taste

Instructions:

1. Place the quinoa in a medium pot and cover with water. Bring to a boil, then reduce heat and simmer for 15 minutes, or until quinoa is tender. Drain and set aside.

2. Heat the oil in a large skillet over medium heat.

3. Add the garlic and cook until fragrant, about 1 minute.

4. Add the cooked quinoa and the remaining ingredients.

5. Stir until combined and season with salt and pepper, to taste.

6. Serve at room temperature or chilled.

Ingredients:

- 2 cans of chickpeas, drained and rinsed

- 2 tablespoons of olive oil

- 1/2 cup of red onion, diced

- 1/2 cup of cucumber, diced

- 1/2 cup of red bell pepper, diced

- 1/4 cup of fresh parsley, chopped

- 2 tablespoons of lemon juice

- Salt and freshly ground black pepper, to taste

Instructions:

1. Place the chickpeas in a large bowl.

2. Heat the oil in a large skillet over medium heat.

3. Add the onion and cook until softened, about 5 minutes.

4. Add the cooked onion, cucumber, bell pepper, and parsley to the bowl with the chickpeas.

5. Drizzle with lemon juice and season with salt and pepper, to taste.

6. Serve chilled or at room temperature.

Ingredients:

- 2 cucumbers, peeled and thinly sliced

- 1/2 cup of plain Greek yogurt

- 2 tablespoons of olive oil

- 1 tablespoon of fresh dill, chopped

- 1 tablespoon of fresh lemon juice

- Salt and freshly ground black pepper, to taste

Instructions:

1. Place the cucumbers in a large bowl.

2. In a small bowl, whisk together the yogurt, olive oil, dill, and lemon juice.

3. Pour the dressing over the cucumbers and toss until evenly coated.

4. Season with salt and pepper, to taste.

5. Chill for at least 30 minutes before serving.

Ingredients:

- 2 tablespoons of olive oil

- 1 medium onion, diced

- 2 cloves of garlic, minced

- 4 cups of gluten-free chicken or vegetable stock

- 4 large carrots, peeled and diced

- 2 tablespoons of fresh ginger, grated

- 1/2 cup of cream

- Salt and freshly ground black pepper, to taste

Instructions:

1. Heat the oil in a large pot over medium heat.

2. Add the onion and garlic and cook until softened, about 5 minutes.

3. Add the stock, carrots, and ginger.

4. Bring to a boil, then reduce heat and simmer until carrots are tender, about 25 minutes.

5. Puree the soup with an immersion blender until smooth.

6. Stir in cream, and season with salt and pepper, to taste.

7. Serve hot.

Ingredients:

- 1 cup of lentils

- 2 cups of water

- 2 tablespoons of olive oil

- 1/4 cup of red onion, diced

- 1/4 cup of fresh parsley, chopped

- 1/4 cup of fresh mint, chopped

- 1/4 cup of fresh lemon juice

- Salt and freshly ground black pepper, to taste

Instructions:

1. Place the lentils in a medium pot and cover with water. Bring to a boil, then reduce heat and simmer for 15 minutes, or until lentils are tender. Drain and set aside.

2. Heat the oil in a large skillet over medium heat.

3. Add the onion and cook until softened, about 5 minutes.

4. Add the cooked lentils and the remaining ingredients.

5. Stir until combined and season with salt and pepper, to taste.

6. Serve at room temperature or chilled.

Ingredients:

- 2 tablespoons of butter

- 1 medium onion, diced

- 2 cloves of garlic, minced

- 5 cups of gluten-free chicken or vegetable stock

- 3 large heads of broccoli, chopped

- 1 cup of cheddar cheese, shredded

- Salt and freshly ground black pepper, to taste

Instructions:

1. Melt butter in a large pot over medium heat.

2. Add the onion and garlic and cook until softened, about 5 minutes.

3. Add the stock and broccoli, and season with salt and pepper.

4. Bring to a boil, then reduce heat and simmer until broccoli is tender, about 25 minutes.

5. Puree the soup with an immersion blender until smooth.

6. Stir in the cheese, and season with salt and pepper, to taste.

7. Serve hot.

Ingredients:

- 2 avocados, diced

- 1/2 cup of cherry tomatoes, halved

- 1/4 cup of fresh parsley, chopped

- 1/4 cup of fresh mint, chopped

- 2 tablespoons of olive oil

- 2 tablespoons of fresh lemon juice

- Salt and freshly ground black pepper, to taste

Instructions:

1. Place the avocados, tomatoes, parsley, and mint in a large bowl.

2. Drizzle with olive oil and lemon juice, and season with salt and pepper, to taste.

3. Toss until combined and chill for at least 30 minutes before serving.

Ingredients:

- 3 apples, diced

- 1/2 cup of dried cranberries

- 1/4 cup of walnuts, chopped

- 2 tablespoons of honey

- 2 tablespoons of olive oil

- 1 tablespoon of fresh lemon juice

- Salt and freshly ground black pepper, to taste

Instructions:

1. Place the apples, cranberries, and walnuts in a large bowl.

2. In a small bowl, whisk together the honey, olive oil, and lemon juice.

3. Pour the dressing over the salad and toss until evenly coated.

4. Season with salt and pepper, to taste.

5. Chill for at least 30 minutes before serving.

1. Gluten-Free Mac and Cheese (30 Minutes)

Ingredients:

-1 pound gluten-free elbow pasta

-4 tablespoons butter

-1/4 cup cornstarch

-2 cups milk

-1 cup shredded cheddar cheese

-Salt and pepper to taste

Instructions:

1. Preheat oven to 375 degrees F and grease a 9-inch baking dish.

2. Cook the pasta in a large pot of salted boiling water according to package instructions.

3. In a saucepan over medium heat, melt the butter and whisk in the cornstarch until combined.

4. Slowly whisk in the milk and bring the mixture to a boil, stirring constantly.

5. Reduce the heat and simmer until the mixture thickens, about 5 minutes.

6. Remove from heat and stir in the cheddar cheese until melted.

7. Drain the cooked pasta and transfer to the prepared baking dish.

8. Pour the cheese sauce over the pasta and stir to combine.

9. Bake for 20 minutes, or until the top is golden brown.

10. Serve hot.

Ingredients:

-1 tablespoon olive oil

-1 cup quinoa, cooked

-1/2 cup diced carrots

-1/2 cup diced celery

-1/2 cup diced onion

-2 cloves garlic, minced

-2 tablespoons gluten-free soy sauce

-1/4 teaspoon ground ginger

-1/4 teaspoon ground black pepper

Instructions:

1. Heat the oil in a large skillet over medium-high heat.

2. Add the quinoa, carrots, celery, onion, and garlic.

3. Cook, stirring occasionally, until the vegetables are tender, about 5 minutes.

4. Add the soy sauce, ginger, and pepper.

5. Cook, stirring frequently, until the quinoa is golden and the vegetables are tender, about 5 minutes.

6. Serve warm.

Ingredients:

-1 pound boneless, skinless chicken breasts, cut into 1-inch cubes

-1/2 cup gluten-free flour

-2 eggs, lightly beaten

-1/2 cup gluten-free bread crumbs

-2 tablespoons olive oil

-Salt and pepper to taste

Instructions:

1. Preheat oven to 375 degrees F and line a baking sheet with parchment paper.

2. Place the chicken cubes in a bowl and season with salt and pepper.

3. Place the flour, eggs, and breadcrumbs in separate shallow dishes.

4. Working in batches, dip the chicken cubes into the flour, then egg, then bread crumbs, making sure to coat each piece completely.

5. Place the coated chicken cubes on the prepared baking sheet.

6. Drizzle with the olive oil and bake for 25 minutes, or until golden brown and cooked through.

7. Serve warm.

Ingredients:

-1 cup grated zucchini

-1/2 cup grated carrots

-1/4 cup gluten-free flour

-2 eggs, lightly beaten

-2 tablespoons olive oil

-Salt and pepper to taste

Instructions:

1. Place the zucchini and carrots in a bowl and season with salt and pepper.

2. Add the flour and eggs and stir until combined.

3. Heat the oil in a large skillet over medium-high heat.

4. Working in batches, scoop 2 tablespoons of the mixture into the pan and flatten into a patty.

5. Cook for 3 minutes per side, or until golden brown and cooked through.

6. Transfer to a plate lined with paper towels to drain.

7. Serve warm.

Ingredients:

-1 pound salmon fillet

-1 tablespoon olive oil

-1/2 teaspoon garlic powder

-1/2 teaspoon onion powder

-1/2 teaspoon dried oregano

-1/2 teaspoon dried thyme

-1/4 teaspoon salt

-1/4 teaspoon ground black pepper

-2 cups mixed vegetables

Instructions:

1. Preheat oven to 400 degrees F and line a baking sheet with parchment paper.

2. Place the salmon on the prepared baking sheet and rub with the olive oil.

3. Sprinkle with the garlic powder, onion powder, oregano, thyme, salt, and pepper.

4. Arrange the vegetables around the salmon.

5. Bake for 20 minutes, or until the salmon is cooked through and the vegetables are tender.

6. Serve warm.

Ingredients:

-4 bell peppers, halved and seeded

-1 cup cooked quinoa

-1/2 cup cooked black beans

-1/2 cup diced tomatoes

-1/2 cup shredded cheese

-1 tablespoon olive oil

-1 teaspoon garlic powder

-1 teaspoon onion powder

-1 teaspoon smoked paprika

-Salt and pepper to taste

Instructions:

1. Preheat oven to 375 degrees F and grease a 9-inch baking dish.

2. Place the bell pepper halves in the prepared baking dish.

3. In a bowl, combine the quinoa, black beans, tomatoes, cheese, olive oil, garlic powder, onion powder, and smoked paprika.

4. Season with salt and pepper.

5. Fill each pepper half with the quinoa mixture.

6. Bake for 25 minutes, or until the peppers are tender and the filling is heated through.

7. Serve warm.

Ingredients:

-4 potatoes, cut into wedges

-2 tablespoons olive oil

-1 teaspoon garlic powder

-1 teaspoon onion powder

-1 teaspoon smoked paprika

-Salt and pepper to taste

Instructions:

1. Preheat oven to 400 degrees F and line a baking sheet with parchment paper.

2. Place the potato wedges on the prepared baking sheet.

3. Drizzle with the olive oil and sprinkle with the garlic powder, onion powder, smoked paprika, salt, and pepper.

4. Toss to combine.

5. Bake for 25 minutes, or until the potatoes are golden brown and crispy.

6. Serve warm.

Ingredients:

-1 pound boneless, skinless chicken breasts

-1/2 cup gluten-free flour

-2 eggs, lightly beaten

-1/2 cup gluten-free bread crumbs

-1/2 cup marinara sauce

-1/2 cup shredded mozzarella cheese

-2 tablespoons olive oil

-Salt and pepper to taste

Instructions:

1. Preheat oven to 375 degrees F and grease a 9-inch baking dish.

2. Place the chicken breasts in a bowl and season with salt and pepper.

3. Place the flour, eggs, and breadcrumbs in separate shallow dishes.

4. Working in batches, dip the chicken breasts into the flour, then egg, then bread crumbs, making sure to coat each piece completely.

5. Place the coated chicken breasts in the prepared baking dish.

6. Drizzle with the olive oil and top with the marinara sauce and mozzarella cheese.

7. Bake for 20 minutes, or until the chicken is cooked through and the cheese is melted and bubbly.

8. Serve warm.

Ingredients:

-4 tilapia fillets

-2 tablespoons olive oil

-1/2 teaspoon garlic powder

-1/2 teaspoon onion powder

-1/4 teaspoon dried oregano

-1/4 teaspoon dried thyme

-1/4 teaspoon salt

-1/4 teaspoon ground black pepper

Instructions:

1. Preheat oven to 375 degrees F and line a baking sheet with parchment paper.

2. Place the tilapia fillets on the prepared baking sheet.

3. Drizzle with the olive oil and sprinkle with the garlic powder, onion powder, oregano, thyme, salt, and pepper.

4. Bake for 20 minutes, or until the fish is cooked through and the edges are golden brown.

5. Serve warm.

Ingredients:

-1 pound gluten-free spaghetti

-1 pound ground beef

-1/4 cup gluten-free bread crumbs

-1 egg, lightly beaten

-1/4 cup grated Parmesan cheese

-1/4 teaspoon garlic powder

-1/4 teaspoon onion powder

-1/4 teaspoon dried oregano

-1/4 teaspoon dried thyme

-1/4 teaspoon salt

-1/4 teaspoon ground black pepper

-1 jar marinara sauce

Instructions:

1. Cook the spaghetti according to package instructions.

2. Meanwhile, in a large bowl, combine the ground beef, bread crumbs, egg, Parmesan cheese, garlic powder, onion powder, oregano, thyme, salt, and pepper.

3. Shape the mixture into 1-inch meatballs.

4. Heat the marinara sauce in a large saucepan over medium heat.

5. Add the meatballs and simmer for 20 minutes, or until cooked through.

6. Drain the cooked spaghetti and transfer to a large serving bowl.

7. Add the meatballs and sauce and toss to combine.

8. Serve warm.

1. Baked Zucchini Fries (15 minutes)

Ingredients:

-2 large zucchini

-¼ cup gluten-free all-purpose flour

-2 eggs

-½ cup gluten-free breadcrumbs

-¼ cup grated Parmesan cheese

-1 teaspoon garlic powder

Instructions:

1. Preheat oven to 400 degrees F. Line a baking sheet with parchment paper.

2. Cut the zucchini into strips and place them in a medium bowl.

3. In a separate bowl, mix together the flour, eggs, breadcrumbs, Parmesan cheese, and garlic powder.

4. Dip the zucchini strips into the egg mixture and then into the breadcrumb mixture, coating them evenly.

5. Place the zucchini strips on the baking sheet and bake for 15 minutes or until golden brown.

Ingredients:

-1 pound asparagus, trimmed

-2 tablespoons olive oil

-1 teaspoon garlic powder

-Salt and pepper, to taste

Instructions:

1. Preheat oven to 400 degrees F. Line a baking sheet with parchment paper.

2. Place the asparagus on the baking sheet and drizzle with olive oil.

3. Sprinkle with garlic powder, salt, and pepper.

4. Bake for 15 minutes or until tender.

3. Sweet Potato Fries (25 minutes)

Ingredients:

-2 sweet potatoes, cut into thin strips

-2 tablespoons olive oil

-1 teaspoon garlic powder

-Salt and pepper, to taste

Instructions:

1. Preheat oven to 400 degrees F. Line a baking sheet with parchment paper.

2. Place the sweet potato strips on the baking sheet and drizzle with olive oil.

3. Sprinkle with garlic powder, salt, and pepper.

4. Bake for 25 minutes or until golden brown and crispy.

Ingredients:

-1 pound fresh green beans, trimmed

-2 tablespoons olive oil

-1 teaspoon garlic powder

-Salt and pepper, to taste

Instructions:

1. Preheat oven to 400 degrees F. Line a baking sheet with parchment paper.

2. Place the green beans on the baking sheet and drizzle with olive oil.

3. Sprinkle with garlic powder, salt, and pepper.

4. Bake for 20 minutes or until tender.

Ingredients:

-1 large butternut squash, cut into cubes

-2 tablespoons olive oil

-1 teaspoon garlic powder

-Salt and pepper, to taste

Instructions:

1. Preheat oven to 400 degrees F. Line a baking sheet with parchment paper.

2. Place the butternut squash cubes on the baking sheet and drizzle with olive oil.

3. Sprinkle with garlic powder, salt, and pepper.

4. Bake for 35 minutes or until tender.

Ingredients:

-1 head broccoli, cut into florets

-2 tablespoons olive oil

-1 teaspoon garlic powder

-Salt and pepper, to taste

Instructions:

1. Preheat oven to 400 degrees F. Line a baking sheet with parchment paper.

2. Place the broccoli florets on the baking sheet and drizzle with olive oil.

3. Sprinkle with garlic powder, salt, and pepper.

4. Bake for 15 minutes or until tender.

Ingredients:

-2 sweet potatoes, cut into ½-inch thick rounds

-2 tablespoons olive oil

-1 teaspoon garlic powder

-Salt and pepper, to taste

Instructions:

1. Preheat oven to 400 degrees F. Line a baking sheet with parchment paper.

2. Place the sweet potato rounds on the baking sheet and drizzle with olive oil.

3. Sprinkle with garlic powder, salt, and pepper.

4. Bake for 30 minutes or until golden brown and crispy.

Ingredients:

-1 pound carrots, cut into 1-inch thick slices

-2 tablespoons olive oil

-1 teaspoon garlic powder

-Salt and pepper, to taste

Instructions:

1. Preheat oven to 400 degrees F. Line a baking sheet with parchment paper.

2. Place the carrot slices on the baking sheet and drizzle with olive oil.

3. Sprinkle with garlic powder, salt, and pepper.

4. Bake for 20 minutes or until tender.

Ingredients:

-2 sweet potatoes, cut into wedges

-2 tablespoons olive oil

-1 teaspoon garlic powder

-Salt and pepper, to taste

Instructions:

1. Preheat oven to 400 degrees F. Line a baking sheet with parchment paper.

2. Place the sweet potato wedges on the baking sheet and drizzle with olive oil.

3. Sprinkle with garlic powder, salt, and pepper.

4. Bake for 25 minutes or until golden brown and crispy.

Ingredients:

-1 pound parsnips, cut into 1-inch thick slices

-2 tablespoons olive oil

-1 teaspoon garlic powder

-Salt and pepper, to taste

Instructions:

1. Preheat oven to 400 degrees F. Line a baking sheet with parchment paper.

2. Place the parsnip slices on the baking sheet and drizzle with olive oil.

3. Sprinkle with garlic powder, salt, and pepper.

4. Bake for 25 minutes or until tender.

1. Gluten-Free Vanilla Cupcakes (20 minutes)

Ingredients:

-1 cup gluten-free flour

-1 teaspoon baking powder

-¼ teaspoon salt

-¼ cup softened butter

-½ cup sugar

-2 eggs

-1 teaspoon vanilla

-½ cup milk

Instructions:

1. Preheat the oven to 350°F and line a cupcake tin with paper liners.

2. In a medium bowl, sift together the gluten-free flour, baking powder, and salt.

3. In a separate bowl, cream together the butter and sugar until light and fluffy.

4. Beat in the eggs one at a time.

5. Stir in the vanilla.

6. Alternate adding the dry ingredients and the milk, beginning and ending with the dry ingredients, and stirring until just combined.

7. Divide the batter among the cupcake liners and bake for 18-20 minutes, or until a toothpick inserted into the center of one of the cupcakes comes out clean.

8. Let cool before frosting with your favorite gluten-free frosting.

Ingredients:

-1 cup gluten-free flour

-1 teaspoon baking soda

-½ teaspoon salt

-¼ cup softened butter

-¼ cup sugar

-½ cup brown sugar

-1 egg

-1 teaspoon vanilla

-1 cup chocolate chips

Instructions:

1. Preheat the oven to 350°F and line a baking sheet with parchment paper.

2. In a medium bowl, sift together the gluten-free flour, baking soda, and salt.

3. In a separate bowl, cream together the butter and sugars until light and fluffy.

4. Beat in the egg and vanilla.

5. Stir in the dry ingredients until just combined.

6. Fold in the chocolate chips.

7. Drop the cookie dough by tablespoonfuls onto the prepared baking sheet.

8. Bake for 12-15 minutes, or until the edges are lightly golden.

9. Let cool on the baking sheet for 5 minutes before transferring to a wire rack to cool completely.

Ingredients:

-1 cup gluten-free flour

-½ teaspoon baking powder

-¼ teaspoon salt

-¼ cup cocoa powder

-½ cup softened butter

-1 cup sugar

-2 eggs

-1 teaspoon vanilla

-½ cup semi-sweet chocolate chips

Instructions:

1. Preheat the oven to 350°F and grease an 8x8" baking pan.

2. In a medium bowl, sift together the gluten-free flour, baking powder, salt, and cocoa powder.

3. In a separate bowl, cream together the butter and sugar until light and fluffy.

4. Beat in the eggs one at a time.

5. Stir in the vanilla.

6. Alternate adding the dry ingredients and the chocolate chips, beginning and ending with the dry ingredients, and stirring until just combined.

7. Spread the batter in the prepared pan and bake for 25-30 minutes, or until a toothpick inserted into the center comes out clean.

8. Let cool before cutting into squares.

Ingredients:

-3-4 apples, peeled, cored, and sliced

-½ cup packed brown sugar

-1 teaspoon ground cinnamon

-¼ teaspoon ground nutmeg

-½ cup gluten-free flour

-½ cup rolled oats

-½ cup softened butter

Instructions:

1. Preheat the oven to 350°F and grease an 8x8" baking pan.

2. Place the apples in the prepared pan.

3. In a small bowl, mix together the brown sugar, cinnamon, and nutmeg.

4. Sprinkle the mixture over the apples.

5. In a medium bowl, stir together the flour, oats, and butter until the mixture is crumbly.

6. Sprinkle the crumble mixture over the apples.

7. Bake for 40-45 minutes, or until the apples are tender and the top is golden brown.

8. Let cool before serving.

Ingredients:

-1 cup gluten-free graham cracker crumbs

-¼ cup butter, melted

-2 8-ounce packages cream cheese, softened

-2 eggs

-1 cup sugar

-1 teaspoon vanilla

Instructions:

1. Preheat the oven to 350°F and grease an 8x8" baking pan.

2. In a small bowl, mix together the graham cracker crumbs and melted butter.

3. Press the mixture into the bottom of the prepared pan.

4. In a medium bowl, beat together the cream cheese, eggs, sugar, and vanilla until smooth.

5. Pour the mixture over the crust.

6. Bake for 45-60 minutes, or until the center is set.

7. Let cool before cutting into bars.

Ingredients:

-1 cup gluten-free flour

-1 teaspoon baking powder

-¼ teaspoon baking soda

-¼ teaspoon salt

-3 ripe bananas, mashed

-½ cup melted butter

-1 cup sugar

-2 eggs

-1 teaspoon vanilla

Instructions:

1. Preheat the oven to 350°F and grease a 9x5" loaf pan.

2. In a medium bowl, sift together the gluten-free flour, baking powder, baking soda, and salt.

3. In a separate bowl, mix together the mashed bananas, melted butter, sugar, eggs, and vanilla until smooth.

4. Stir in the dry ingredients until just combined.

5. Pour the batter into the prepared pan.

6. Bake for 55-60 minutes, or until a toothpick inserted into the center comes out clean.

7. Let cool before slicing.

Ingredients:

-1 10-ounce package marshmallows

-3 tablespoons butter

-4 cups gluten-free rice cereal

Instructions:

1. Grease an 8x8" baking pan.

2. In a large saucepan, melt together the marshmallows and butter over low heat, stirring constantly until the mixture is smooth.

3. Remove from heat and stir in the rice cereal.

4. Press the mixture into the prepared pan and let cool before cutting into squares.

Ingredients:

-1 cup gluten-free flour

-1 teaspoon baking powder

-½ teaspoon baking soda

-¼ teaspoon salt

-2 eggs

-½ cup melted butter

-1 cup sugar

-½ cup cocoa powder

-1 teaspoon vanilla

-½ cup milk

Instructions:

1. Preheat the oven to 350°F and grease two 9" round cake pans.

2. In a medium bowl, sift together the gluten-free flour, baking powder, baking soda, and salt.

3. In a separate bowl, beat together the eggs, melted butter, sugar, cocoa powder, and vanilla until light and fluffy.

4. Alternate adding the dry ingredients and milk, beginning and ending with the dry ingredients, and stirring until just combined.

5. Divide the batter between the two prepared pans and bake for 40-50 minutes, or until a toothpick inserted into the center of one of the cakes comes out clean.

6. Let cool before frosting with your favorite gluten-free frosting.

9. Gluten-Free Blueberry Pie (60 minutes)

Ingredients:

-2 cups fresh or frozen blueberries

-1/3 cup sugar

-2 tablespoons cornstarch

-1 tablespoon lemon juice

-1 teaspoon vanilla

-1 gluten-free pie crust

Instructions:

1. Preheat the oven to 375°F.

2. In a medium bowl, mix together the blueberries, sugar, cornstarch, lemon juice, and vanilla until combined.

3. Pour the mixture into the prepared pie crust.

4. Bake for 50-60 minutes, or until the filling is bubbly and the crust is golden brown.

5. Let cool before serving.

Ingredients:

-1 cup gluten-free flour

-2 teaspoons baking powder

-¼ teaspoon salt

-¼ cup softened butter

-½ cup sugar

-1 egg

-½ cup milk

-2 cups sliced strawberries

-1 cup heavy cream

-2 tablespoons sugar

Instructions:

1. Preheat the oven to 375°F and line a baking sheet with parchment paper.

2. In a medium bowl, sift together the gluten-free flour, baking powder, and salt.

3. In a separate bowl, cream together the butter and sugar until light and fluffy.

4. Beat in the egg.

5. Alternate adding the dry ingredients and the milk, beginning and ending with the dry ingredients, and stirring until just combined.

6. Drop the dough by tablespoonfuls onto the prepared baking sheet.

7. Bake for 15-20 minutes, or until the tops are lightly golden.

8. In a medium bowl, whip together the heavy cream and sugar until stiff peaks form.

9. Serve the shortcakes topped with the sliced strawberries and whipped cream.